Stir Crazy Through the Lens of Chaos
Cabin Fever, Island Fever, and the Rest
Your 38th Psychiatric Consultation
William R. Yee M.D., J.D.,
Copyright Applied for Sept. 3rd, 2023

ISBN 978-1-304-88408-4

I want to thank Lisa Guzman for asking about the use of Chlorpromazine-Thorazine.

I rely on Chlorpromazine-Thorazine because:
1. I have long experience with Chlorpromazine-Thorazine;
2. I find Chlorpromazine-Thorazine covers the entire spectrum of Temporary Insanity treated in Emergency Room Settings and Acute Care Psychiatric Hospitals including but not limited to:
  a. homicidal
  b. suicidal
  c. grave disability
  d. schizophrenia spectrum disorders
  e. bipolar mania,

f. agitated states

g. anger

3. The medical research does not identify any antipsychotic as superior to Chlorpromazine-Thorazine for Temporary Insanity states that I treat.

4. Chlorpromazine has a wide dosing range and can be titrated up rapidly.

5. I find that Chlorpromazine is more effective for Temporary Insanity as described above than Haldol, Seroquel, and Zyprexa.

6. Chlorpromazine does not have the excessive QTc risk of Geodon-Ziparsodone, Haldol-Haloperidol, or Seroquel-Quetiapine:

   a. ++ Moderate >9 to <16 milliseconds
      Chlorpromazine ++

   b. +++ Severe >16 milliseconds
      Haloperidol +++
      Ziprasidone +++
      Quetiapine +++
      Thioridazine +++
      Methadone +++

7. By using Thorazine Equivalents after the acute phase is over Chlorpromazine is easily cross titrated to any other antipsychotic agent or mood stabilizer,

8. The most important issue to address in Temporary Insanity as described above is aggression with injury to self or others.
   a. I find that Chlorpromazine is the most consistently effective medication for acute aggression based upon my experience.
   b, Sleep after an initial oral dose of Chlorpromazine effectively stops Aggression.
   c. The, "Thorazine Shuffle," is part of the Initial effect of Thorazine and indicates a calm state unlikely to result in assault in most cases.

Currently the cost of Chlorpromazine is inflated in the United States by the practices of the Pharmaceutical Industry and Heavy Lobbying in the Government.

A solution would be to have state agencies band together to manufacture generic medications or in the alternative to purchase psychotropic drugs offshore along with masks and ventilators.

Now let us review the available literature that supports my observations and practice of starting with Chlorpromazine-Thorazine as the first choice when treating Temporary Insanity due to mental illness.

Chlorpromazine is listed as a WHO essential medication.

Chlorpromazine was developed in 1950 and was the first antipsychotic on the market. It is on the World Health Organization's List of Essential Medicines. Its introduction has been labeled as one of the great advances in the history of psychiatry.
Chlorpromazine - Wikipedia

Chlorpromazine replaced the Lobotomy.

Thus, the disparaging moniker, "Chemical Lobotomy."

Chlorpromazine has fallen out of favor in the United States and now is expensive, despite being the first antipsychotic medication and the replacement for the Frontal Lobe Lobotomy.

However, WHO lists chlorpromazine as a basic and essential medication that should be available in all health care settings.

I rely on:
Wikipedia
https://en.wikipedia.org › wiki › Chlorpromazine.

"The WHO essential medicines list (EML) is a register of minimum medicine needs for every health-care system (Bloom, 2011). The basic concept is that high priority drugs should be available as part of a functioning health system at all times for all people, guiding physicians to evidence-based and rational prescribing."

I rely on:
What is the WHO essential medicines list?
M. Purgato and C. Barbui
Epidemiol Psychiatr Sci. 2012 Dec; 21(4): 343–345.
Published online 2012 Jul 30. doi: 10.1017/S204579601200039X
PMCID: PMC6998134
PMID: 22846155

Chlorpromazine's indications include:
1. Schizophrenia (primarily the positive symptoms)
2. Acute manic type of manic-depressive illness
3. Acute agitation marked by explosive hyperexcitable behavior out of proportion to the initial provocation
4. To control nausea and vomiting, including intraoperative nausea and vomiting, (part of drug withdrawal).

5. Persistent singultus (chronic hiccups)
6. Relief of apprehension before surgery
7. Adjunct treatment of tetanus
8. Acute intermittent porphyria
9. Adjunct treatment of serotonin syndrome (off-label)
10. Migraine associated relief of nausea and vomiting (off-label)

I rely on:
Chlorpromazine
Sukhmanjeet Kaur Mann; Raman Marwaha.
Last Update: May 16, 2023.
https://www.bap.org.uk/articles/chlorpromazine-the-first-antipsychotic/

Bookshelf ID: NBK553079PMID: 31971720

In the United States the FDA has approved Chlorpromazine for the treatment of:
1. schizophrenia; to control nausea and vomiting; 2. or relief of restlessness and apprehension before surgery;
3. psychosis due to acute intermittent porphyria;
4, as an adjunct in the treatment of tetanus;
5. to control the manifestations of the manic type of manic-depressive illness.
6. for relief of intractable hiccups.
7. for the treatment of severe behavioral problems in children (1 to 12 years of age) marked by combativeness and/or explosive hyperexcitable behavior (out of proportion to immediate provocations), and
8. the short-term treatment of hyperactive children who show excessive motor activity with accompanying conduct disorders consisting of some or all the following symptoms:
    a. impulsivity,
    b. difficulty sustaining attention,
    c. aggressivity,
    d. mood lability, and
    e. poor frustration tolerance.

I rely on:
Chlorpromazine Prescribing Information
Package insert/product label
Generic name: chlorpromazine
hydrochloride
Dosage form: injection
Drug classes: Phenothiazine antiemetics,
Phenothiazine antipsychotics
Chlorpromazine was originally assessed as an anesthetic prior to its use as an antipsychotic agent.

Clients on Chlorpromazine may not feel pain with acute appendicitis.

Thus, Clients on chlorpromazine may not experience pain with a ruptured appendix, resulting in perforated appendix, peritonitis, and death.

Clients withdrawing from Fentanyl Often prefer chlorpromazine as it reduces pain experienced during Fentanyl withdrawal.

"Laborit observed that chlorpromazine induced calmness without sedation when given to patients prior to surgery and this led him to suggest it may be of use in psychiatry."

This calm may be related to suppression of Frontal Lobe Executive function and the Thorazine Shuffle described above. Since clients are generally on a gurney prior to surgery, the Thorazine Shuffle would not be observed.

I rely on:
Chlorpromazine, the first antipsychotic medication: history, controversy and legacy
Peter Haddad, Robert Kirk, and Richard Green
31st October 2016 ·

I rely on:
BMJ Open. 2017; 7(9): e017150.
Published online 2017 Sep 25. doi: 10.1136/bmjopen-2017-017150
PMCID: PMC5623499
PMID: 28951411
Perforated appendicitis in patients with schizophrenia: a retrospective cohort study
Yoshimasa Nishihira,1 Rita L McGill, and Mitsuyo Kinjo

The cause of most mental illness is not known. An exception is psychosis with Acute Intermittent Porphyria. Although it is known that the psychotic episode is caused by porphyria, the precise pathway is not known.

However, chlorpromazine was initially the drug of choice for relieving the psychosis of Acute intermittent porphyria.

As early as 1956 it was determined that a single dose of 100mg of Thorazine or 25mg of Thorazine three or four times a day is sufficient to resolve the pain and psychosis of Acute Intermittent Porphyria.

I rely on:

ACUTE INTERMITTENT PORPHYRIA - RELIEF OF SEVERE PAIN AFTER

TREATMENT WITH CHLORPROMAZINE
HYDROCHLORIDE
Report of a Case ALFRED M. TAYLOR, M.D.
Cleveland Clinic Quarter;y
Volume 29, October 1962

And

Acute Intermittent Porphyria Presenting
Solely with Psychosis: A Case Report and
Discussion
Bharat Kumar, M.D.

Psychosomatics 2012:53:494–498 © 2012 The
Academy of Psychosomatic Medicine.
Published by Elsevier Inc. All rights
reserved.

It is postulated that hallucinations,
delusions, and paranoia of schizophrenia
are due to hyperactivity of dopamine at D_2
dopamine receptors in the mesolimbic
pathway of the brain. Thorazine binds to
those receptors.

D_2 stimulators (agonists) include opiates,
alcohol, nicotine, amphetamines, and

cocaine. The use of opiates, alcohol, amphetamines, and cocaine is associated with psychotic episodes and aggression.

It is speculated that the flat affect, lack of psychosocial motivation and engagement, and other negative symptoms of schizophrenia may be due to under stimulation of the D_1 receptors.

I am accustomed to treating the most severely mentally ill, e.g. Suicidal, Homicidal, and Gravely disabled. That is the criteria for admission to an Acute Care Psychiatric Hospital or an Emergency Medical Center for triage to an Acute Care Psychiatric Hospital.

Chlorpromazine is effective for Bipolar Mania, Schizophrenia, Schizoaffective Disorder, Aggression in Adults and Children, Agitation Associated with Pain, and it can be rapidly titrated up by oral or intramuscular administration.

Geodon-Ziprasidone and Haldol are less effective for aggression and bipolar disorder than Chlorpromazine based upon my personal experience.

Geodon and Haldol have the additional burden of high QTc risk.

Clozaril was released to the market after a six-week study demonstrated that it was able to reduce symptoms by 20% in 30% of clients refractory to haldol and other clients,

Due to the slow titration Clozaril is not suitable for acute care hospitals which often have an average length of stay of less than a week.

Let us look at the QTc intervals of some of the psychotropic medications commonly used.

QTc intervals above 450 are associated with Torsades de Pointes, Ventricular Fibrillation, and sudden death.
I recently placed a patient on Abilify 5mg BID because of a QTc of 485.
Psychotropic drugs often increase the QTc.
Psychotropics that do not increase the QTc are rated as 0= none
Aripiprazole NR= Not Reported
Paliperidone ER NR= Not Reported
Lithium NR= Not Reported
Nortriptyline NR= Not Reported

Sertraline NR= Not Reported
Fluvoxamine NR= Not Reported
Duloxetine NR= Not Reported
Reboxetine NR= Not Reported
Excitalopram NR= Not Reported

Methylphenydate NR= Not Reported
Atomoxetine NR= Not Reported

Valproate NR= Not Reported
Lamotrigine NR= Not Reported
Biperidine NR= Not Reported
Olanzapine NR= Not Reported

+ Mild = >5 to<9 milliseconds increase
Perphenazine +
Fluphenazine +
Clozapine +
Risperidone +

Mirtazapine +
Trazodone +
Mirtazapine +
Trazodone +
Venlafaxine +
Citalopram +
Bupropion +
Imipramine +
Desipramine +
Chloral Hydrate +

++ Moderate >9 to <16 milliseconds
Chlorpromazine ++
Fluoxetine ++
Amitriptyline ++
Doxepine ++

+++ Severe >16 milliseconds
Haloperidol +++
Ziprasidonen +++
Quetiapinen +++
Thioridazine +++
Methadone +++

Thorazine is the standard against which other psychotropic medications are measured.
Other psychotropic are measured in Chlorpromazine Equivalents.
Generic Brand Dose Equivalent to 100mg of Chlorpromazine-Thorazine
First Generation Antipsychotics
ChlorpromazineThorazine©.................100 mg
FluphenazineProlixin©.........................2 mg
HaloperidolHaldol©...............................2 mg
LoxapineLoxitane©...............................10 mg
PerphenazineTrilafon©.........................8 mg
PimozideOrap©.......................................2 mg
ProchlorperazineCompazine©..............15 mg
TrifluoperazineStelazine©....................2-5 mg

ThioridazineMellaril©...........................100 mg
ThiothixeneNavane©................................4 mg
Second Generation Antipsychotics
AripiprazoleAbilify©..............................7.5 mg
AsenapineSaphris©...................................4 mg
ClozapineClozaril...................................100 mg
IloperidoneFanapt©..............................3-4 mg
LurasidoneLatuda©................................16 mg
OlanzapineZyprexa©..................................5 mg
PaliperidoneInvega©................................2 mg
QuetiapineSeroquel©.............................75 mg
RisperidoneRisperdal©...........................1 mg
ZiprasidoneGeodon©...............................60 mg

I rely on:
Psychiatric Pharmacy Essentials:
Antipsychotic Dose Equivalents
Reviewer 1: Krina Patel, PharmD, BCPP
Reviewer 2: Carly Rainey, PharmD, BCPS
Reviewer 3: Joseph M. Cusimano, PharmD,
BCPP
2022-2023 AAPP Resident and New
Practitioner Committee
The American Association of Psychiatric
Pharmacists (AAPP)
055 O Street
Suite S113
Lincoln, NE 68510
T: 402-476-1677

info@aapp.org
https://aapp.org/guideline/essentials/antipsy
chotic-dose-equivalents

Stir Crazy, Cabin Fever, Island Fever, Rumspringa (not insanity but scheduled abnormal behaviors), Amok, Berserk, can be classified as forms of temporary insanity.

They meet in the psychiatric hospital where the criteria for admission are suicidal, homicidal, and gravely disabled, which are also forms of temporary insanity.
The human brain is composed of, "100 billion neurons and 10× more glial cells."

I rely on:
The Human Brain in Numbers: A Linearly Scaled-up Primate Brain
Suzana Herculano-Houzel
Front Hum Neurosci. 2009; 3: 31.
Published online 2009 Nov 9. Prepublished online 2009 Aug 5.
doi: 10.3389/neuro.09.031.2009
PMCID: PMC2776484
PMID: 19915731

The human brain is a self-organizing system.

A self-organizing system is, "a core concept of Systems Science. It refers to the ability of a class of systems (self-organizing systems (SOS)) to change their internal structure and/or their function in response to external circumstances."

I rely on:
Banzhaf, W. (2009). Self-organizing Systems . In: Meyers, R. (eds) Encyclopedia of Complexity and Systems Science. Springer, New York, NY. https://doi.org/10.1007/978-0-387-30440-3_475

It is postulated that schizophrenia can be caused by pathological pruning of the brain creating independent partitions of the brain that are self-organizing. This results in random partitions. An emergent symptom in the schizophrenic patient is the inability of the patient to perceive random physical and psychological functions as part of his or herself.

The inability to recognize parts of one's body or intellectual and emotional processes is called anosognosia.

For a deeper look at these concepts, I refer the reader to:
Schizophrenia
A Diagnosis Looking for a Cause and a Cure
Your Seventh Psychiatric Consultation
William Yee M.D., J.D.
Copyright Applied for 01/19/2020.

For the present consider the mechanism of action of antipsychotic agents.

"First-generation antipsychotics are dopamine receptor antagonists (DRA) and are known as typical antipsychotics. Second-generation antipsychotics are serotonin-dopamine antagonists and are also known as atypical antipsychotics."

I rely on:
Antipsychotic Medications
Krutika Chokhawala; Lee Stevens.
StatPearls [Internet].
Copyright © 2023, StatPearls Publishing LLC.
Bookshelf ID: NBK519503PMID: 30137788
https://www.ncbi.nlm.nih.gov/books/NBK519503/
Last Update: February 26, 2023.

Altering dopamine and serotonin-dopamine receptor activity does not join dependent self-organizing symptoms into a single self-organizing system.

Antipsychotic medication is more like giving aspirin for pneumonia than giving an antibiotic for pneumonia.

Antipsychotic medications do not cure schizophrenia.

Examine the, "Post by Former NIMH Director Thomas Insel: Antipsychotics: Taking the Long View," By Thomas Insel on August 28, 2013.

Thomas R. Insel, M.D is credible by virtue of the fact that he was Director of the National Institute of Mental Health (NIMH) from 2002-2015.

The literature and the pharmaceutical industry warn of a decline in function with each psychotic break. Dr. Insel points to facts that suggest moderation in the use of antipsychotic medication for the best results.

Dr. Insel pointed out the fact that patients that were treated with antipsychotics and had a six-month remission and stopped the antipsychotics had a functional recovery rate of 40.4 percent after seven years.

Dr. Insel pointed out the fact that patients that were treated with antipsychotics had a six-month remission, and continued the antipsychotics had a functional recovery rate of only 17.6 percent after seven years.

Dr. Insel points out that a functional recovery is often better served by stopping the antipsychotic medications and focusing on alternative treatments.

Altering dopamine and serotonin-dopamine receptor activity has value during and acute psychotic episode.

However, altering dopamine and serotonin-dopamine receptor activity is only a small part of the puzzle of schizophrenia and not as relevant to a long-term functional recovery as alternative treatments.

Examine the work of Anne Sullivan.

Anne Sullivan's work with Helen Keller would be the kind of treatment intervention necessary to connect the separate islands of neurons.

Ann Sullivan was Helen Keller's nanny and worked with Hellen Keller from the time she got up in the morning until she went to bed at night. This is continuous, one on one treatment.

This is the kind of intervention you see occurring between mother and child during the first few years of life.

It is a matter of making the child or the patient aware of the thousands of connections among thoughts, emotions, physical experiences, memories, social expectations, communications skills which are necessary for a functional personality in the local culture.

This is labor intensive and not compatible with current models that focus on brief therapies in the office and in the hospital.

Let us look at temporary insanity.

Stir Crazy, Cabin Fever, Island Fever, Rumspringa, Amok, Berserk, Danger to Self, Danger to others, and grave disability can all be classified as temporary insanity.

Danger to Self, Danger to Others, and Grave Disability are required for admission to a psychiatric hospital. Less severe mental illness may be safely treated in less restrictive settings such as a doctor's office.

Stir crazy is defined as, "any person who has become restless, agitated, or anxious from being or feeling entrapped in some place."
Source
Merriam-Webster
Publishing company
https://www.merriam-webster.com/dictionary/stir-crazy

In prisons in Michigan in 1987 prisoners would label it as, "going on a nut," and other phrases. I listened to prisoners who told me they would, 'bop till they drop," meaning they would hit their heads on the wall until they felt high from a concussion.

Cabin Fever, Island Fever, Rumspringa, Amok, Berserk, Danger to Self, Danger to others, and grave disability can all be classified as temporary insanity.

Cabin Fever is defined as, "the feeling of being angry and bored because you have been inside for too long," Cambridge Dictionary.

Island Fever is defined as,
"A psychological illness that usually affects poor people found in Hawaii and other islands.
Island Fever is the realization that you are stuck on whichever island you are living and not going anywhere."
Urban Dictionary
https://www.urbandictionary.com › define › term=Isla.

Rumspringa, "Amish teenagers may be encouraged to explore otherwise forbidden or strictly regulated behaviors before making the choice to commit to the church." Strictly speaking this is not temporary insanity. But it is a temporary major change of behavior.

Berserk:
adjective
violently or destructively frenzied; wild; crazed; deranged: He suddenly went

berserk.
noun
Scandinavian Legend.
Also ber·serk·er. an ancient Norse warrior who fought with frenzied rage in battle, possibly induced by eating hallucinogenic mushrooms.
ORIGIN OF BERSERK
C19: Icelandic berserker, from björn bear + serkr shirt

Amok,
noun
(among members of certain Southeast Asian cultures) a psychic disturbance characterized by depression followed by a manic urge to murder.
adjective
amuck.
ORIGIN OF AMOK
C17: from Malay amoq furious assault

Mass Shootings,
"Mass shooting," also called active shooter incident, as defined by the U.S. Federal Bureau of Investigation (FBI), an event in which one or more individuals are "actively engaged in killing or attempting to kill people in a populated area. Implicit in this definition is the shooter's use of a firearm."
https://www.britannica.com/topic/mass-shooting
The Editors of the Encyclopaedia Britannica
This article was most recently revised and updated by Pat Bauer.

Suicide by Cop.
"When a suicidal individual provokes a law enforcement officer into killing him or her."
Suicide by Cop: A Psychiatric Phenomenon
Ralph H. de Similien, M.D., M.S., M.Ed., Adamma Okorafor, M.D.
Published Online:26 Jan 2017https://doi.org/10.1176/appi.ajp-rj.2017.120107

To appreciate Temporary Insanity, one should read about feral children. These children would not be affected by culture during episodes of temporary insanity.

8 Children Who Were Raised by Animals
By Bryan Nelson
Bryan Nelson
SUNY Oswego
University of Houston
Updated November 10, 2019
8 Children Who Were Raised by Animals
By Bryan Nelson
Updated November 10, 2019

Temporary insanity is shaped by culture. A kind culture will create a kind insanity and a psychopathic culture will create a psychopathic insanity.

Let us examine self-organizing systems through the lens of Chaos Theory.

Self-Organizing Systems are sets of individual elements that all follow a few simple rules. By operation of these few simple rules the system self organizes.

The brain can function like a self-organizing system and have periods of stability alternating with periods of instability. These states can be strongly influenced by a single factor.

"Complex systems such as the environment, economy and government often function more effectively if there are only a number of simple rules in place that allow for orderly and self-organizing behaviour to emerge,"

I rely on:
Simple rules and self-organization: A complex systems' perspective on South Africa's COVID-19 response
Christo Coetzee
Jamba. 2021; 13(1): 1013.
Published online 2021 May 13. doi: 10.4102/jamba.v13i1.1013
PMCID: PMC8182558
PMID: 34191987

For this reason, I encourage clients to utilize a number of alternatives to medications to improve the periods of stability. These changes have the potential to make future periods of stability better for the patient and those around the patient. The list includes, but is not limited to the following:

a. Meditation to improve depression, anxiety, and concentration.;
b. Aerobic Exercise and Diet to improve

depression, anxiety and physical health.

c. Breathing and Muscle Relaxation for control of stress and anxiety.

d. Building a Support System for Quality of Life.

e. Using Kindness to deploy the Golden Rule to make friends who respond with kindness.

f. Cognitive Behavior Therapy to make positive changes.

g. Symptom substitution such as replacing addiction to drugs with addiction to exercise, addiction to learning, addiction to reading, addiction to work, etc.

h. Imagination exercises such as imagining yourself feeling good about yourself and the world around you.

i. Learning to live with a cup half full, for example exploiting your skills and opportunities and enjoying what you have and not wasting time being unhappy about what you don't have.

j. Use of a day planner as a medical journal to track
   i. sleep, eating, exercise stress, anxiety, depression and other issues.
   ii. Listing things that make the day better and strategies to make these things a larger part of your life.
   iii. listing things that make your day

worse and strategies to make these
things a smaller part of your life.
iv. make small daily changes to make
your life better so that you can look
forward to having a better life every
day for the rest of your life.

"For example, an attractor that describes a
system that cycles periodically over the
same set of states, never coming to rest, is
known as a limit cycle."

I rely on:
Simple rules and self-organization: A
complex systems' perspective on South
Africa's COVID-19 response
Christo Coetzee
Jamba. 2021; 13(1): 1013.
Published online 2021 May 13. doi:
10.4102/jamba.v13i1.1013
PMCID: PMC8182558
PMID: 34191987
https://www.ncbi.nlm.nih.gov/pmc/articles/P
MC8182558/

Finally, let us look at how to filter
information from, "published medical
research."

There are many issues to consider.

The Crisis in Science

There has been a crisis in science for decades. Scientific research that is published can't be reproduced by other scientists. Unless the research can be reproduced, it is not sound science. 1,500 scientists lift the lid on reproducibility.

I rely on:
Monya Baker nature news feature article
Published: 25 May 2016
Nature volume 533, pages452–454 (2016)

The crisis in scientific publications is getting worse. Interesting research is more likely to be published if it is interesting even if it is not science that can be replicated by other scientists.

"Papers that cannot be replicated are cited 153 times more because their findings are interesting, according to a new UC San Diego study."

I rely on:
A New Replication Crisis: Research that is
Less Likely to be True is Cited More
May 21, 2021, | By Christine Clark
https://ucsdnews.ucsd.edu/pressrelease/a-
new-replication-crisis-research-that-is-less-
likely-be-true-is-cited-
more?fbclid=IwAR3Eiqlm-
hdMJTZ70FnhLv8WpMg5WrGTvnvX5aIlwx
75dB4Qt OQon4jlnA

If a healthcare professional does not have
the correct information, how is informed
choice even possible?

> Misinformation provided by
> pharmaceutical companies.

It seems that all businesses and
multinational corporations tend to promote
bad science in support of their revenue
streams and narratives.

The welfare of the public is a secondary
consideration for the purposes of window
dressing and deflection.

I rely on:

Trial sans Error: How Pharma-Funded
Research Cherry-Picks Positive Results
Clinical trial data on new drugs is
systematically withheld from doctors and
patients, bringing into question many of the
premises of the pharmaceutical industry—
and the medicine we use.
By Ben Goldacre on February 13, 2013,
Published by Faber and Faber, Inc. © 2013.
Ben Goldacre. Scientific American
https://www.scientificamerican.com/article/
trial -sans-error-how-pharma-funded-
research-cherry-picks-positive-results/

"The boundaries between academic
medicine - medical schools, teaching
hospitals, and their faculty - and the
pharmaceutical industry have been
dissolving since the 1980s, and the
important differences between their
missions are becoming blurred. Medical
research, education, and clinical practice
have suffered as a result."

I rely on:

Ex-editor of NEJM tells how Big Pharma has corrupted academic institutions.
In the May/June issue of the Boston Review, Dr. By Susan Perry

The physician is often misinformed by the medical literature for a variety of reasons.

First there is publication bias.

Publication bias

For a fact check and deeper look I refer the reader to:

Publication bias in meta-analyses from the Cochrane Database of Systematic Reviews
Michal Kicinski David A. Springate
Evangelos
Kontopantelis
First published: 18 May 2015
https://doi.org/10.1002/sim.6525

For more information I refer the reader to:

Not to be confused with Reporting bias or Media bias. Publication bias is a type of bias that occurs in published academic research. It occurs when the outcome of an experiment or research study influences the decision whether to publish or otherwise distribute it. Publishing only results that show a significant finding disturbs the balance of findings and inserts bias in favor of positive results.[1] The study of publication bias is an important topic in metascience. Studies with significant results can be of the same standard as studies with a null result with respect to quality of execution and design.[2] However, statistically significant results are three times more likely to be published than papers with null results.[3] A consequence of this is that researchers are unduly motivated to manipulate their practices to ensure that a statistically significant result is reported.[4]
From Wikipedia, the free encyclopedia

I will leave it to the reader to research the following list of flaws in research regarding the risks and benefits of psychotropic medications.

Research fails to include pregnant women and children on ethical grounds.
Research fails to include the elderly and people with multiple medical problems.
Research fails to include people on multiple medications.
Small sample size is not sufficient to provide reliable data.
Samples are not random because they do not include people who refuse.
Samples are not random because populations may not be accessible.
Studies are not randomized.
Studies are not blinded.
Studies do not use the same criteria for diagnosis or target symptoms.
The studies are of short duration.
Studies do not clearly separate spontaneous remission from medication effect.
Studies do not account for cognitive dissonance in addition to placebo effect.
It is difficult to identify altered data, "fudging."

This is not even the tip of the iceberg. One study uncovered 710 unique research flaws for excluding research from evidence-based databases.

For fact checking and a deeper look at the shortcomings of medical research I refer the reader to:
A Large-Scale Analysis of the Reasons Given for Excluding Articles that are Retrieved by Literature Search During Systematic Review Tracy Edinger, ND, MCR and Aaron M. Cohen, MD, MS AMIA Annu Symp Proc. 2013; 2013: 379–387. Published online 2013 Nov 16.
PMCID: PMC3900186
PMID: 24551345

And also:
Addicting Medications, No Functional Recovery
The Long View
Your Nineteenth Psychiatric Consultation
William R. Yee M.D., J.D.
Copyright Applied for January 1st, 2021

It is difficult for the physician to wade through extensive medical literature and weed out the truth from the false research results being published.

"Considering that these surveys ask sensitive questions and have other limitations, it appears likely that this is a conservative estimate of the true prevalence of scientific misconduct."
I refer the reader to:

How Many Scientists Fabricate and Falsify Research? A Systematic Review and Meta-Analysis of Survey Data
Daniele Fanelli
Published: May 29, 2009
https://doi.org/10.1371/journal.pone.0005738
and:
Prevalence of Research Misconduct and Questionable Research Practices:
A Systematic Review and Meta-Analysis
Yu Xie, Kai Wang & Yan Kong
Practices: A Systematic Review and Meta-Analysis. Sci Eng Ethics 27, 41 (2021).
https://doi.org/10.1007/s11948-021-00314-9
August 10, 2018

"Findings

In this systematic review of 265 studies comprising 400 647 drug samples and meta-analysis of 96 studies comprising 67 839 drug samples, the prevalence of substandard and falsified medicines in low- and middle-income countries was 13.6% overall (19.1% for antimalarials and 12.4% for antibiotics). Data on the estimated economic impact were limited primarily to market size and ranged widely from $10 billion to $200 billion."

I refer the reader to:
Prevalence and Estimated Economic Burden of Substandard and Falsified Medicines in Low- and Middle-Income Countries A Systematic Review and Meta-analysis
Sachiko Ozawa, PhD, MHS1,2; Daniel R. Evans, MSc2; Sophia Bessias, MPH3; et al Deson G. Haynie, MHS4; Tatenda T. Yemeke, MSc; Sarah K. Laing, MPH2; James E.
Herrington, PhD5
JAMA Netw Open. 2018;1(4): e181662. doi:10.1001/jamanetworkopen.2018.1662

"Both publication bias and outcome reporting bias may affect meta-analyses, and the effect can be unpredictable. Adding unreported data from both published and unpublished drug trials to 41 meta-analyses caused 46% of the meta-analytic effect estimates to show lower efficacy of the drug, 7% to show identical efficacy, and 46% to show greater efficacy."

I refer the reader to:
Preferred reporting items for systematic review and meta-analysis protocols (PRISMA-P) 2015: elaboration and explanation
Larissa Shamseer, David Moher, Mike Clarke,
Davina Ghersi, Alessandro Liberati (deceased), Mark Petticrew, Paul Shekelle, Lesley A Stewart7the PRISMA-P Group
BMJ 2015; 349 doi:
https://doi.org/10.1136/bmj.g7647
(Published 02 January 2015)
Cite this as: BMJ 2015;349:g7647

My final thoughts on massive doses of antipsychotic medications.

Recently I recommended that a patient be sent to an emergency room for triage and admission to a medical hospital for intensive care for side effects of polypharmacy.

Polypharmacy raises serious risks of neuroleptic malignant syndrome, serotonin syndrome, atropine toxicity, multiple organ failure, and death.

Massive doses of antipsychotic medications provide marginal or no benefit for the treatment of psychosis.

In 2000 Kapur et al. determined that

1, 65% D2 saturation by Haldol achieved a therapeutic response,

2. 72% saturation by Haldol raised prolactin levels and

3. 78% saturation by Haldol precipitated extrapyramidal side effects.

4. raising saturation above 65% did not appear to yield additional benefit.

5. 2.5mg a day of Haldol achieved 65% to 75% D2 occupancy.

6. They recommended a starting dose of two or three milligrams a day.

D_2 saturation above 65% does not appear to provide additional benefits in reducing psychotic symptoms and only causes gynecomastia with lactation in both men and women and at higher levels, Tardive Dyskinesia, (EPS).

The lowest effective dose is the best practice.

Exceeding the lowest effective dose appears to cause serious side effects without a benefit according to research published as early as 2000.

I rely on:
See, "Relationship Between Dopamine D 2 Occupancy, Clinical Response, and Side Effects: A Double-Blind PET Study of First-Episode Schizophrenia," Shitij Kapur, M.D., Ph.D., F.R.C.P.C., Robert Zipursky, M.D., F.R.C.P.C., Corey Jones, B.A., Gary Remington, M.D., Ph.D., F.R.C.P.C., and Sylvain Houle, M.D., Ph.D., F.R.C.P.C. Am J Psychiatry 157:4, April 2000

As the Baby Boomers hit the wall and enter nursing homes and hospitals in large numbers it will be necessary to start weaning them off medications they have been taking for many years for many medical conditions.

This is because with age the physiologic reserves decline.

A measure of physiologic reserves is the LD50. The LD50 is the amount of stress that the body can tolerate before 50% of the stressed population dies. The elderly are more likely to die from flu or Covid than healthy adults. The LD50 is lower for the elderly than healthy young adults.

A red flag for this is the Black Box Warning for sudden death with the use of antipsychotics in the elderly with dementia. "The FDA asked manufacturers to place a "black box" warning on drug labels—indicating an adverse reaction that may result in death or serious injury-noting the increased death rates and that 'these drugs are not approved for the treatment of behavioural symptoms in elderly patients with dementia."

I rely on:
American Geriatrics Society 2023 updated AGS Beers Criteria® for potentially inappropriate medication use in older adults
By the 2023 American Geriatrics Society Beers Criteria® Update Expert Panel
First published: 04 May 2023
https://doi.org/10.1111/jgs.18372
It is malpractice and elder abuse to add medications to the elderly if the side effects of medications outweigh the benefits.

It is malpractice and elder abuse not to wean the elderly off medications with side effects that cause falls, loss of memory, impaired frontal lobe executive functions and sudden death.

For a clear understanding of the issues that underly the need to reduce the elderly I refer the reader to:

"The American Geriatrics Society (AGS) Beers Criteria® (AGS Beers Criteria®) for Potentially Inappropriate Medication (PIM) Use in Older Adults is widely used by clinicians, educators, researchers, healthcare administrators, and regulators. Since 2011, the AGS has been the steward of the criteria and has produced updates on a

regular cycle. The AGS Beers Criteria® is an explicit list of PIMs that are typically best avoided by older adults in most circumstances or under specific situations, such as in certain diseases or conditions."
American Geriatrics Society 2023 updated AGS Beers Criteria® for potentially inappropriate medication use in older adults

Journal of the American Geriatrics Society Volume 71, Issue 7, July 2023, Pages 2052-2081
By the 2023 American Geriatrics Society Beers Criteria® Update Expert Panel
First published: 04 May 2023
https://doi.org/10.1111/jgs.18372
I must end this missive at some point, and I choose to end it here and now.

I am here to do no harm and help if I can. Thank you for your time and attention.

Be kind and you can be my friend.

William R. Yee M.D., J.D.
Board Certified Psychiatrist.
Practicing Medicine and Psychiatry without interruption since 1972 in Michigan, Indiana, Kentucky, California, Texas, and now in Alaska at your service.

"Pre-Existing text," includes names of symptoms and medical illnesses, medications, people, corporations, law cases, statutes, text of statutes, the titles of articles and books, the content of articles and books cited, FDA Labels and FDA releases and images taken from the internet.

My copyright claim is a claim to the "original text," which is my personal experience as described in the text and my commentary on names of symptoms and medical illnesses, medications, people, corporations, law cases, statutes, text of statutes, the titles of articles and books, the content of articles and books cited, FDA Labels and FDA releases and images taken from the internet.

Coda: The Long View:
Copy Right Applied for October 29, 2023

The reader is advised that the most
important recent research is the following:
A. pharmacotherapy does not change
     brain activity or connectivity
B. Psychotherapy alters neural
 activities and connectivity of
    C. regions serving
        1. executive control
        2. emotion regulation
        3. dialectical behavior therapy and
        4. psychodynamic therapies are the
          most effective.

Hallucination like experiences and
delusions are common in
individuals without psychoses.

Every hallucination, every delusion, and
every paranoia should NOT be treated.

I refer the reader to:
Studying Healthy Psychosis like
Experiences to Improve Illness Prediction
Philip R. Corlett, PhD, Sonia Bansal, PhD
James M. Gold, PhD

Published Online: March 8, 2023
Special Communication

A. Moral Intuitions
   1. I would not want this for myself.
   2. Treatment is making my patient suffer horribly.
   3. There is no good option here.
   4. No matter what I do, I don't think my patient is going to get better.
   5. I have no choice but to use coercion.
   6. I feel that we're only making matters worse.
   7. I would not be surprised if my patient died this year.
B. Thoughts and feelings like these are Associated with
   1. unease
   2. helplessness
   3. being stuck
C. are common among mental health care professionals
D. especially those caring for persons
   1. with severe and persistent mental illness (SPMI)
E. Typically, these concerns are
   1. dismissed or
   2. attributed to burnout
   3. lack of training or

4. lack of experience, or

5. unprofessional pessimism.

F. Examine these thoughts through the
   lens of moral intuition.

   1. with the potential

   2. to improve care

   3. of persons living with SPMI.

G. In some cases the pursuit of
   rehabilitative goals is futile.

1. some have advocated palliative
   approaches to mental health care

2. the overarching palliative goal in
   mental health care is to

   a. maximize quality of life

   b. through harm reduction

   c. relief of suffering

I refer the reader to:
Moral Intuitions About Futility as Prompts
for Evaluating Goals in
Mental Health Care
AMA Journal of Ethics
Published Online: September 1, 2023

The Covid Pandemic has altered physical
and mental health in the general
population that requires this addition to my
prior publication.

Recent advances in MRI's, Genetics, DNA knowledge, and medical technology in general require this addition to my prior publications.

There are ethical issues that impinge on the practice of psychiatry.

One author asks how a psychiatrist should conduct himself when:
1. There is limited time for CBT motivationally enhanced therapy?
2. Are there significant side effects of antipsychotics?
3. The client's cognitive functions are impaired.

The author does not provide explicit answers, but merely asks questions that are easily asked but without answers that satisfy anyone.

I refer the reader to:
Should Antipsychotics' Risks Be Accepted by Clinicians on Behalf of Patients to Achieve Benefits of Mitigating Older Adults' Behavioral Symptoms in Short-Staffed Units?
Alex Rollo MD, Jena Kar DO, Uma

Suryadevara MD et al?
AMA Journal of Ethics
Published Online: October 1, 2023

A. Mental illness accounts for almost
   1. 30% of disease burden
2. among noncommunicable diseases
B. Environmental factors account for approximately
   1. 50% of the attributable risk for mental Disorder
C. Environmental factors that are shared among groups, such as
   1. urbanicity,
   2. climate and
   3. pollution,
   4. regional socioeconomic status,
   5. shared psychosocial stressors, s
   6. such as the COVID-19 pandemic
   7. are less well investigated

I refer the reader to: Addressing Global Environmental Challenges to Mental Health Using Population Neuroscience A Review JAMA Psychiatry Published Online: August 23, 2023

Borderline Personality Disorder
1. No class of psychoactive medication is consistently effective
2. No medications is FDA approved for Borderline Personality Disorder
3. Pharmacotherapy is not recommend for Treatment of any core symptom of BPD
   A. marked emotional instability
   B. transient stress-related paranoid ideation
4. Functional magnetic resonance imaging studies have convincedly demonstrated
   A. pharmacotherapy does NOT change brain activity or connectivity, /
   B. Psychotherapy
1. ALTERS neural activities and
2. ALTERS connectivity of
   C. regions serving
      1. executive control
      2. emotion regulation
      3. dialectical behavior therapy and
      4. psychodynamic therapies are
effective.

I rely on:
Review of Borderline Personality Disorder
Falk Leichsenring, DSc; Nikolas Heim, MA, MSc3; Frank Leweke, MD1; et al

JAMA Published Online: February 28, 2023
Review

The prevalence of depression is
1. 5% in the general population
2. 10% low socioeconomic position (SEP)

Depression is known to be higher in identified populations:
1. 27% chronic obstructive pulmonary disease (COPD) has been 2.
2. 20% type 2 diabetes,
3. 20% myocardial infarction
4. 17% cancer, to 17%
5. 33%. stroke
6, 27% women who experienced intimate partner violence
7. 2-fold increased risk of depression in people with lower SEP.16

The COVID-19 pandemic and its containment measures have profound adverse effects.

The COVID-19–related stressors include but are not limited to:
1. loss of employment
2. illness or death of a relative

3. reduced access to mental health services
4. frequent concerns about mental and physical health
5. 29% of health care staff suffered emotional distress
6. depression
7. anxiety-related disorders
8. Suicide

The stress of the Covid Pandemic increased depression among the population and the most at risk were those suffering from Sequelae of:
1. physical or psychological abuse
2. mental health conditions
3. preexisting physical health conditions
4. low social support
5. low socioeconomic position (SEP)

I refer the reader to:
Levels of Severity of Depressive Symptoms Among At-Risk Groups in the UK During the COVID-19 Pandemic
Eleonora Iob, MSc Philipp Frank, MSc Andrew Steptoe, DSc et al
JAMA Network Open
Published Online: October 26, 2020
Original Investigation

Long Covid is chronic Covid symptoms
A. 13.9% of those who had tested positive
   for COVID-19,
B. 1.7% of US adults
C. age above 40 years have greater risk
D. Female greater risk
E. Multiple Organ Systems:
   1. respiratory,
   2. metabolic,
   3. cardiovascular,
   4. gastrointestinal, and
   5. neuropsychiatric
F. Symptoms include but are not limited to
   1. fatigue was most common
   2. loss of smell
   3. "brain fog"
   4. shortness of breath
   5. poor memory
   6. cognitive symptoms
   7. anxiety
   8. sleep disruption

I refer the reader to:
Prevalence and Correlates of Long COVID
Symptoms Among US Adults
Roy H. Perlis, MD, MSc.
Mauricio Santillana, Phd.
Katherine Ognyanova, PhD. et al
JAMA Network Open

Published Online: October 27, 2022
Original Investigation

Schizophrenia
A. can create a high disease burden for
   some patients.
B. Schizophrenia is often refractory to
   multiple interventions.
C. 34% of schizophrenia is treatment-
   resistant schizophrenia.
D. 4.9% of people with schizophrenia die by
   suicide.
E. 6% of disability benefits recipients had
   schizophrenia or other psychotic
   disorder
F. Beneficence: the best interests standard.
 1. First: weighing the benefits
    and burdens
 2. Second: is it good enough?
 3. Third: moral and legal duties

I refer the reader to:
What Makes Palliative Mental Health Care
Ethical Health Care?
Virginia A. Brown; Ashley Trust
AMA Journal of Ethics
Published Online: September 1, 2023

However, healthcare in jails and prisons is slow to change.

Estelle v. Gamble held that failure to provide adequate medical
care to incarcerated people because of deliberate indifference
violates the Eighth Amendment's prohibition against cruel and unusual punishment.

What does that mean for the health care practitioner?
1. "deliberate indifference" and
2. "serious medical need" are subject to judicial interpretation.

The health care practitioner and chain of command for health care in correctional facilities must
A. guess as to the scope of their liabilities
B. guess as to the scope of their authority

Regarding the provision of health care in correctional facilities:
A. All such decisions are subject to judicial review and this patient population tends to be litigious.

However, the courts have determined that, "serious medical need" does include:
A. the threat of death
B. degeneration
C. extreme pain
D. suicidal tendencies
E. withdrawal symptoms.

Courts have ruled that
A. symptoms without an accompanying diagnosis
B. do not constitute a
C. "serious medical need."

The practitioner is faced with the question of what to do:
A. when the complexity of the case
B. does not allow a diagnosis
C. Ganser's Syndrome?
D. Malingering?
F. Factitious Disorder?

I refer the reader to:
Health Care in U.S. Correctional Facilities - A Limited and Threatened Constitutional Right
Marcella Alsan, M.D., Ph.D., M.P.H., Crystal S. Yang, J.D., Ph.D., James R. Jolin, Lucy Tu, and Josiah D. Rich, M.D., M.P.H.

March 2, 2023
N Engl J Med 2023; 388:847-852
DOI: 10.1056/NEJMms2211252

In 2004 the literature did not raise red flags
for the use of psychotropic medications
in the presence of renal failure.
A. Renal failure is common.
B. Renal Failure often has comorbid
   psychiatric illness.
C. Renal failure can require
D. adjustments to medications.

E. One author concluded that
1. psychotropic medications were safely
   used with renal failure

I refer the reader to:
Update on psychotropic medication use in
renal disease
Lewis M Cohen 1, Edward G Tessier,
Michael J Germain, Norman B Levy
PMID: 14709759 DOI:
10.1176/appi.psy.45.1.34
Psychosomatics. 2004 Jan-Feb;45(1):34-48.
doi: 10.1176/appi.psy.45.1.34.

Covid changed that and reminds us how important it is to keep up with the rapid advances of medicine and evidenced based medical care.

1. Chronic kidney disease (CKD) is common
2. affects almost all organ systems
3. impairs quality of life.

CKD (Chronic Kidney Disease) is caused by:
1. diabetes mellitus,
2. hypertension,
3. tubulointerstitial diseases,
4. glomerulonephritis,
5. polycystic kidney diseases,
6. obstructive uropathy
7. congenital kidney malformations

.

CKD, manifests with:
1. progress decline in eGFR (estimated glomerular filtration rate)
2. appetite loss
3. nausea
4. vomiting
5. fatigue
6. lethargy
7. muscle cramps,

8. edema of limbs
9. itching
10. insomnia
11. hypertension
12. dyspnea
13. chest pain,
14. altered urine output.
15. altered behavior,
16. altered lifestyle
17. poor medication adherence

I refer the reader to:
Management of Psychiatric Disorders in Patients with Chronic Kidney Diseases.
Dalal PK, Kar SK, Agarwal SK.
Indian J Psychiatry. 2022 Mar;64(Suppl 2):S394-S401. doi:
10.4103/indianjpsychiatry.indianjpsychiatry_1016_21. Epub 2022 Mar 23.
PMID: 35602366; PMCID: PMC91221

Haloperidol is considered safe in renal disease.
The kidneys are not involved in the metabolism and excretion of haloperidol.

I refer the reader to:
When to adjust the dosing of psychotropics in patients with renal impairment

Current Psychiatry. 2016 August;15(8):60-66
By Sarah Ward, PharmD Julius Paul
Roberts, DO William J. Resch DO,
DFAPA Christopher Thomas, PharmD,
BCPS, BCPP
SAVY PSYCHOPHARMACOLOG

When considering QTc prolongation the
following risks have been identified.

Second generation antipsychotics
1, Highest risk: ziprasidone and
   iloperidone
2. Lowest risk: aripiprazole and lurasidone

FDA warnings (black box)
1. Ziprasidone
2. Quetiapine
3. Intravenous haloperidol

Both first- and second-generation
antipsychotics have been linked to:
1. ventricular arrhythmias
2. sudden cardiac death.

Increased risk:
1. haloperidol
2. prochlorperazine
3. thioridazine

4. quetiapine
5. risperidone

FDA black box warning for
1. second-generation antipsychotics
2. in elderly patients with dementia

Antipsychotics not associated with QT prolongation are:
A. lurasidone;
B. cariprazine; and
C. brexpiprazole.

I refer the reader to:
The Risk of QTc Interval Prolongation with Psychotropics
Christopher M. Celano, MD, FACLP
Associate Director, Cardiac Psychiatry Research Program
Massachusetts General Hospital Assistant Professor of Psychiatry, Harvard Medical School
October 22, 2020
https://mghcme.org/app/uploads/2020/10/Celano-Academy-Course-QTc-2020.pdf

And:
Chohan PS, Mittal R, Javed A.
Antipsychotic Medication and QT

Prolongation. Pak J Med Sci. 2015 Sep-Oct;31(5):1269-71. doi: 10.12669/pjms.315.8998. PMID: 26649027; PMCID: PMC4641296.

1. quetiapine is the optimal antipsychotic drug
2. for the treatment of patients with delirium and
3. prolonged baseline QTc intervals.

I refer the reader to:
Comparison of Antipsychotics for the Treatment of Patients With Delirium and QTc Interval Prolongation: A Clinical Decision Analysis
Ken Kurisu Kazuhiro Yoshiuchi
Front. Psychiatry, 25 June 2021
Sec. Psychopharmacology
Volume 12 - 2021

A. Adults older than 64
B. had an almost 2-fold increase in hospitalization.
C. For AKI within the next 90 days who received.
1. quetiapine
2. risperidone
3. olanzapine

Antipsychotics not associated with QT prolongation are:
A. lurasidone;
B. cariprazine; and
C. brexpiprazole.

As a general rule, if the QTc is significantly
A. prolonged (>500 ms)
B. . with no other reversible causes
C. The following psychotropics should be
 Used
  1. lurasidone;
  2. cariprazine; and
  3. brexpiprazole.

I refer the reader to:
Antipsychotics Linked to Acute Kidney
Injury
Deborah Brauser
August 19, 2014

Bipolar disorder
A. 8 million cases in the United States
B. recurrent episodes
 1. of depression and
2. mania or hypomania.
C. depression is the most frequent initial presentation.
D. 75% of symptomatic time consists of depression.
E. treatment is often delayed for years.
1. long-term treatment consists of mood stabilizers,
     a. lithium
     b. valproate
     c. lamotrigine.
2. antipsychotic agents with side effects
     a. quetiapine
     b. aripiprazole
     c. asenapine
     d. lurasidone
     e. cariprazine,
F. Antidepressants are not recommended as monotherapy.
1. More than 50% of bipolar disorder patients are medication noncompliant.
2. Life is reduced 12 to 14 years

3. 2-fold increase in cardiovascular Mortality.
4. Prevalence comorbidities:
a. metabolic syndrome (37%),
b. obesity (21%),
c. cigarette smoking (45%), and
d. type 2 diabetes (14%) are
e. annual suicide rate is approximately 0.9%
f. 15% to 20% of people with bipolar disorder die by suicide.

I refer the reader to:
Diagnosis and Treatment of Bipolar Disorder: A Review
Nierenberg AA, Agustini B, Köhler-Forsberg O, Cusin C, Katz D, Sylvia LG, Peters A, Berk M. JAMA. 2023 Oct 10;330(14):1370-1380. doi: 10.1001/jama.2023.18588. PMID: 37815563.
I refer the reader to:
Diagnosis and Treatment of Bipolar Disorder: A Review
Nierenberg AA, Agustini B, Köhler-Forsberg O, Cusin C, Katz D, Sylvia LG, Peters A, Berk M. JAMA. 2023 Oct 10;330(14):1370-1380. doi: 10.1001/jama.2023.18588. PMID: 37815563.

A. Recently completed study resolves schizophrenia's complex pathobiology
1. genetic studies
2. implicate genes localizing to hippocampal glutamatergic neurons
3. loss-of-function mutations in subunits of
   a. α-amino-3-hydroxy-5-methyl-4-isoxazolepropionic acid (AMPA)
   b. N-methyl-d-aspartate (NMDA) glutamate receptors,
B. Functional and structural magnetic resonance imaging (MRI)
   1. Support anatomical findings of genetics
   2. localizing to the hippocampus and
   3. its CA1 subdivision as the brain region affected by schizophrenia.
C. The pathophysiology of the disordered hippocampus emerges from
   1. functional imaging and
   2. magnetic resonance spectroscopy (MRS).
D the disordered hippocampus is characterized by
   1. abnormal increases in glutamate

levels
2. hyperactivity
3. atrophy
E. Clinically, schizophrenia is characterized by both
1. positive symptoms
  a. psychosis and
2. negative symptoms
  b. cognitive deficits
F. Support ofthe hippocampal pathophysiological state is
1. linked to glutamate receptor loss of function
2. and can drive schizophrenia's symptoms
G. provided by medical conditions.
1. that phenocopy schizophrenia's symptoms
  a. paraneoplastic limbic encephalitis
  b. caused by antibodies directed against either the
    i. hippocampal-enriched AMPA or NMDA receptors
2. neurotoxic syndromes induced by an overdose of drugs that inhibit the
  a. hippocampal-enriched NMDA Receptors
  b. and seizures that
    i. localize to thehippocampus and

ii emanate from the hippocampus.
c. helping to explain this clinical
   phenocopy and
   i. how it links to schizophrenia's
   genetic triggers
   ii. inhibiting hippocampal
   glutamate receptors
   iii. in mice
 d. causes hippocampal
    i. glutamate elevation
    ii. hyperactivity and
    iii. atrophy
H. Hippocampal hyperactivity
   1. can drive striatal dopamine release.
   2. via monosynaptic connections
      with the striatum
   3. explaining positive symptoms, and
   4. hippocampal atrophy.
   5. can partly explain the disorder's
      negative symptoms
I. Future MRS studies can be used to
   1. test the hypothesis for
   2. why glutamate is abnormally elevated
   3. in the hippocampus of patients
   4. with schizophrenia and
   5. related disorders.
J. More importantly,
   1. an MRS signature of pathway
      dysfunction

2. can be used to accelerate the discovery of
3. clinically meaningful interventions
4. for devastating lifelong brain disorders
5. that emerge in adolescence.

I refer the reader to:
Why Hippocampal Glutamate Levels Are Elevated in Schizophrenia
Jia Guo, PhD1;
Douglas L. Rothman, PhD2;
Scott A. Small, MD1
JAMA Psychiatry
Published Online: January 25, 2023
Neuroscience and Psychiatry

I am here to do no harm and help if I can.

Thank you for your time and attention.

Be kind and you can be my friend.

William R. Yee M.D., J.D.
Board Certified Psychiatrist.
Practicing Medicine and Psychiatry without interruption since 1972 in Michigan, Indiana, Kentucky, California, Texas, and now in Alaska at your service.

"Pre-Existing text," includes names of symptoms and medical illnesses, medications, people, corporations, law cases, statutes, text of statutes, the titles of articles and books, the content of articles and books cited, FDA Labels and FDA releases and images taken from the internet.

My copyright claim is a claim to the "original text," which is my personal experience as described in the text and my commentary on names of symptoms and medical illnesses, medications, people, corporations, law cases, statutes, text of statutes, the titles of articles and books, the content of articles and books cited, FDA Labels and FDA releases and images taken from the internet.

The Clozaril Controversy
Copyright Applied for 11/03/2023

Fact Check and Predict the Road To Wisdom.
There is a Crisis in Science,
Pharmaceutical Companies Pay for Research to Sell Their Drugs
Clozaril is a Dangerous Drug.
The Evidence that Supports the Advantages of Clozaril is Sketcchy.
The Evidence that Supports the Risk of Clozaril is masked ieht "Optimism?"
I Predict that at the End of the Day Clozaril will be placed into the bin with Thalidomide and Lobotomies.
Overvalued, Overutilized, and another Failed Medical Experiment.

Ask Frances Oldham Kelsey, MD, PhD what she thinks about Clozaril?

Frances Oldham Kelsey, MD, PhD, then 96 and frail, was chaperoned by her two daughters for the occasion. She beamed as FDA leaders honored her in speeches before presenting her with the Dr. Frances O. Kelsey Award for Excellence and Courage in Protecting the Public Health.

How a courageous physician-scientist saved the U.S. from a birth-defects catastrophe
March 9, 2020
Written By Stephen Phillips

Clozapine is a dangerous medication with marginal benefits and inconsistent evidence supporting its use.
It is expensive to prescribe and manage.
Its cost will deprive patients of alternative treatments.
Recent advances in technology confirms the fact that psychotherapy alters connections in the brain that reflect changes in thinking and behavior,
Recent advances in technology reveal the fact that antipsychotic medications do not alter connections in the brain that reflect changes in thinking and behavior,
There is a crisis in science,
Part of that crisis is that the pharmaceutical industry pays for research to promote the sale of their products.
Government agencies that rely on Clozaril are at risk of spending alot of money with limited, no or a negative benefit at the end of the day.
I rely on my 50 years of experience in psychiatry and the following information.

Fact Check and Predict the Road to
Wisdom.

There is a Crisis in Science.

Pharmaceutical Companies Pay for
Research to Sell Their Drugs.

Clozaril is a Dangerous Drug.

The Evidence that Supports the Advantages
of Clozaril is Sketchy.
The Evidence that Supports the Risk of
Clozaril is masked by "Optimism?"

I Predict that at the End of the Day
Clozaril will be placed into the bin with
Thalidomide and Lobotomies.
Overvalued, Overutilized, and another
Failed Medical Experiment.

Ask Frances Oldham Kelsey, MD, PhD what
she thinks about Clozaril?

Frances Oldham Kelsey, MD, PhD, then 96
and frail, was chaperoned by
her two daughters for the occasion.

She beamed as FDA leaders honored her in speeches before presenting her with the Dr. Frances O. Kelsey Award for Excellence and Courage in Protecting the Public Health.

How a courageous physician-scientist saved the U.S. from a birth-defects catastrophe
March 9, 2020
Written By Stephen Phillips

Clozapine is a dangerous medication with marginal benefits and inconsistent evidence supporting its use.

It is expensive to prescribe and manage.

Its cost will deprive patients of alternative treatments.

Recent advances in technology confirm the fact that psychotherapy alters connections in the brain that reflect changes in thinking and behavior.

Recent advances in technology reveal the fact that antipsychotic medications do not alter connections in the brain that reflect changes in thinking and behavior.

There is a crisis in science.

Part of that crisis is that the pharmaceutical industry pays for research to promote the sale of their products.

Government agencies that rely on Clozaril are at risk of spending a lot of money with limited, no, or a negative benefit at the end of the day.

I rely on my 50 years of experience in psychiatry and the following information.

Efficacy and safety of clozapine in psychotic disorders - a systematic quantitative meta-review.
Wagner, E., Siafis, S., Fernando, P. et al.
Transl Psychiatry 11, 487 (2021).
https://doi.org/10.1038/s41398-021-01613-2

Clozapine "best evidence" for use.
1. Efficacy
2. Effectiveness
3. tolerability.

Management of
1. clozapine and

2. clozapine-related adverse events
PRISMA-conforming quantitative meta-review of Primary outcome effect sizes

1. relative risk ratios (RR) and
2. standardized mean differences (SMD).
The AMSTAR-2 checklist.

Of the 112 meta-analyses included in our review,
61 (54.5%) had AMSTAR-2 high quality
Clozapine superior effects on
1. Positive,
2. negative, and
3. overall symptoms and relapse rates
4. in schizophrenia
5. compared to first-generation
   antipsychotics (FGAs) and to
6. Pooled FGAs/second-generation
   antipsychotics (SGAs) in treatment-resistant schizophrenia (TRS).

Despite an unfavorable metabolic and hematological adverse-event profile compared to other antipsychotics,
1. hospitalization,
2. mortality and
3. all-cause discontinuation (ACD) rates
4. clozapine surprisingly shows a pattern of

superiority.
5. beneficial efficacy outcomes in
6. bipolar disorder and
7. Parkinson's disease psychosis (PDP).

Furthermore, we grouped outcomes into
1. short-term (up to 12 weeks),
2. medium-term (13–26weeks), and
3. long-term (over 26 weeks).

Clozapine "appears" to be superior to FGAs
in RCTs(short, medium, and long-term)
with small to medium effects sizes

Clozapine "appears" to be superior to
risperidone in Japanese populations with a
medium effect size [29, 31].

For TRS, clozapine "appears" to be
1. not significantly superior to pooled SGAs
in observational studies [82],
2. not significantly superior to other single
SGAs [100] in RCTs.
3. When FGAs/SGAs are pooled, clozapine
appears to be superior in
improving positive symptoms in RCTs in
TRS with a small effect size

Negative symptoms in schizophrenia
1. Clozapine is "not" superior to SGAs in observational studies
2. Clozapine "is" superior to most FGAs in RCTs
3. with both small and large effect sizes
4. "except" short-term data vs "Chlorpromazine."
5. There is "conflicting evidence" regarding the superiority of clozapine vs. Pooled SGAs in TRS
6. clozapine "appears" "inferior" to Quetiapine (short-term, only 2 studies with n total = 142) with medium effect sizes.
7. clozapine "appears" "inferior" to aripiprazole medium-term in RCTs with a small effect size.

Overall symptoms in schizophrenia
Clozapine "appears" to be:
1. superior to "placebo" in short-term RCTs With large effect sizes.
2. superior to FGAs in RCTs with small to medium effect sizes
3. superior to SGAs in observational studies with a small effect size
4. superior to quetiapine in long-term RCTs with a large effect size

For TRS, clozapine "appears" to be superior to
1. CPZ with a medium effect size
2. superior vs. mixed FGAs/SGAs in RCTs with small effect sizes
_+_+_+_+_+_+_+
3. but the evidence is suggestive that clozapine is "not superior vs. Other Antipsychotics in long-term RCTs."
_+_+_+_+__+_+_+

Other efficacy measures in schizophrenia
Clozapine has a favorable profile in terms of dropout due to inefficacy compared to
1. placebo with a large effect size
2. CPZ with a medium effect size
3. SGAs, namely risperidone with medium effect sizes
4. and in terms of ACD compared to FGAs with small effect sizes grouped SGAs in observational studies with a small effect size
5. some single SGAs (e.g. risperidone and quetiapine) with small effect sizes

With regard to relapse, clozapine "appears" to be superior to
1. FGAs long-term
2. but "evidence" from meta-analyses is "inconsistent"

With regard to response, clozapine "appears" to be superior to
1. placebo with large effect sizes
2. superior to FGAs short-term with "small effect sizes"
3. but "not superior" to single SGAs (e.g
   1. quetiapine,
   2. risperidone,
   3. olanzapine)

As a second-line agent, clozapine appears to be superior to
1. risperidone and other antipsychotics with small effect sizes
Evidence "does not support superiority" of clozapine for hospitalization rate
1. vs. SGAs
2. reduction of suicide/self-injurious behavior vs. SGAs in observational studies
3. and "does not support superiority" for anti-suicidal effects in long-term RCTs vs.

olanzapine, but

4. meta-analytic evidence from one long
   -term trial showed superior effects of
   clozapine vs. Olanzapine.
5. Meta-analytic evidence suggests superior
   effects of clozapine on "hostility"
   compared to FGAs in RCTs in mixed
   A. short-,
   B. medium-, and
   C. long-term RCTs
   D. with a medium effect size
6. and on
   A. cognition
   B. vs. SGAs in
   C. TRS in observational studies with
   D. a small effect size.
7. whereas mostly "nonsignificant effects"
   on cognition compared to
   A. FGAs and
   B. SGAs were
   C. observed in RCTs
8. and even
   A. inferior effects vs. S
   B. ingle FGAs, e.g. sertindole

With regard to psychosocial functioning, clozapine appears
1. "not" to have significantly more beneficial effects
2. compared to SGAs

For quality of life, available data is scarce

No superior efficacy of clozapine vs. other antipsychotics could be
shown for
1. mania in bipolar disorder short-term
2. For PDP, clozapine seems to be superior vs. quetiapine short-term in terms of clinical global impression with large effect sizes.

Tolerability of clozapine (SMD and RR)
1. Clozapines significantly higher risk for weight gain with small to medium effect sizes
2. increased risk to develop type 2 diabetes
3. significantly fewer EPS or use of antiparkinsonian medication compared to FGAs with small effect sizes
4. SGAs with large effect size and
   A. Especially risperidone with a medium effect size
5. clozapine is associated with a

significantly lower mortality compared to both FGAs and SGAs with small to large effect sizes (due to dropouts?) despite an unfavorable profile regarding
A. sedation/dizziness,
B. Anticholinergic,
C. hematological, and
D. cardiac events,
E. different metabolic outcomes and
F. dropouts due to adverse events

Clozapine appears to be not significantly different from
1. Amisulprid
2. olanzapine,
3. Zotepine
4. risperidone
in terms of overall symptoms.

For TRS, clozapine is presumed to be "not more efficacious than"
1. olanzapine,
2. risperidone or
3. ziprasidone
in the sub analyses including only TRS trials in overall symptoms in the meta-analysis from
Leucht et al. being in linewith the evidence from the meta-analysis from Samara et al.

where also only blinded RCTs were included.

Clozapine was not significantly superior to most other APs with regard to overall symptom reduction

For treatment-resistant positive symptoms, clozapine "seems" to have significantly superior beneficial effects
1. compared to quetiapine and
2. haloperidol on single-substance level,
3. +_+but not compared to olanzapine+_+

When comparators are pooled as a group (FGA + SGA)
Clozapine was shown to have superior effects for treatment-resistant overall and positive symptoms.

Nevertheless, for overall and positive symptoms in TRS,
1. inconsistent evidence is reported in meta-analyses due to differences in study selections, study populations, in the handling of study characteristics, and in methodological approaches

For treatment-resistant negative symptoms, clozapine was shown to be
1. slightly superior to FGAs
2. despite inconsistent results
3. but-according to a large body of evidence
4. not significantly superior in comparison to SGAs
5. if, then only on short-term
6. Nevertheless, negative symptom data did not include a separation of primary from secondary negative symptoms, which hampers interpretability of the results.

For cognition and psychosocial functioning,
1. clozapine is not presumed to be significantly superior compared to other SGAs
2. While evidence for the efficacy of clozapine for first-episode psychosis is scarce
3. limited evidence suggests superior effects for clozapine as a second-line Agent compared to other antipsychotics, such as, e.g. risperidone
Clozapine shows beneficial effects on psychosocial function but
1. without superiority to other antipsychotics
2. Inconclusive results are available for pro

-cognitive effects of clozapine vs.
A. FGAs and
B. SGAs
Clozapine dosages above 400 mg/day, clozapine was
1. superior to risperidone,
2. but not olanzapine and
3. evidence of effects between clozapine standard, low and very low dose regimes
   On overall outcome in schizophrenia is sparse
4. For bipolar disorder, the efficacy of clozapine seems to be similar to other antipsychotics in manic episodes
5. For neurological disorders, the largest body of evidence is available for PDP, Where low-dose clozapine (range from 12.5 to 50 mg) showed beneficial effects
   On psychotic symptoms)
   _+_+_even though negative results are Reported_+_+_+

The results of this meta-review should be interpreted with caution due to the inherent limitations of the meta-analyses and their included studies.

For the above I rely on:

Efficacy and safety of clozapine in psychotic disorders - a systematic quantitative meta-review.
Wagner, E., Siafis, S., Fernando, P. et al.
Transl Psychiatry 11, 487 (2021).
https://doi.org/10.1038/s41398-021-01613-2

I am not a stranger to this conversation. I engaged in a similar conversation about Clozaril in 2016 when a prior meta-analysis found that Clozaril was NOT superior to other antipsychotic medications.

From: Yee, William
Sent: Wednesday, June 22, 2016 10:36 AM
If the inter-rater reliability was in the diagnosis of Schizophrenia with paranoid schizophrenia etc the whole concept is subject to skepticism.
The basis of psychiatric diagnosis is consensus in speculation rather than a genuine grounding in scientific fact.

The concepts of schizophrenia and mood disorders are collections of symptoms floating above a black box that we have yet to penetrate.

Mental illness is not a specific illness like cryptococcus pneumonia, but a fever with the underlying illness yet to be discovered.

From: Johnson, Thomas
Sent: Wednesday, June 22, 2016 10:28 AM
I remember when I was working at UCIMC with Dr. Maguire and Potkin on some research we were in workshops where we all would attend. Shown video of psychotic patients. then we all rated them.
It was like a competition between the various research sites. To see who could have the highest interrater consistency.
I think we need this. It also involved a nice hotel and dinner....

From: Johnson, Thomas
Sent: Wednesday, June 22, 2016 9:43 AM
Maybe this is another separate issue but along the line of Dr. Deane's thinking.
We have received patient's at ASH from CDCR who were initially in the ICU from clozapine induced eosinophilia and peritonitis, I believe the patient also developed some pulmonary clots as a result. NEARLY FATAL.
I remember the patient well he was admitted to Unit 23. In fact one of the

psychiatrists at Patton did a grand rounds in which he was referenced tallking about the risks of Eosinophilia and Clozapine. When the patient arrived here my anxiety was quite high I will admit. What am I going to do with a young man who is refractory to medications and has almost died from clozapine?
Sounds like a real losing battle AND NO WIN SITUATION. Chances are so slim that anything is
really going to help this patient.
RESULTS- HALDOL 5 MG - DID EXTREMELY WELL. MODEL PATIENT. THIS PATIENT
OBVIOUSLY DID NOT NEED CLOZAPINE. I REPEATEDLY HEAR FROM STAFF THAT MANY OF THE PATIENTS WE HAVE ARE NO BETTER THAN THEY WERE 5 YEARS AGO. wHEN THEY WERE ONLY ON HALDOL.
Some of our long time staff know these patients well.
We currently have no mechanism for accurately rating patients level of psychosis PRIOR TO INITIATION OF CLOZAPINE.
We have hospital policies that place the physician and nursing staff at high level of responsibility for the safe administration of

clozapine. Yet repeatedly the policies are not followed. Patients are non compliant with "Showing their feces"
Patients are shoked when they come to the treatment unit and hear we want to see it. tHEY
ACT AS IF THEY HAVE NEVER SHOWED THEIR FECES ON THE PREVIOUS UNIT.
Even our patients who are poor reporters are shocked that we are insisting to see.
We have no PANNS (Positive and Negative Symptoms Scores to reflect on) RESULTS OF TREATMENT
If we are to be cutting edge and using clozapine so agressively we should first have in place a mechanism to determine if the medication has been truly helpful. Otherwise the risks are not
justified.
wE ALSO MAY WANT TO CONSIDER A CLOZAPINE UNIT. IT WOULD BE MUCH EASIER TO
PLACE A BATHROOM MONITOR ON ONE UNIT.
I HAVE ALSO BEEN REMINDED RECENTLY THAT THIS IS A GROUP PRACTICE. WHILE

**THIS IS TRUE, WHO WILL BE
RESPONSIBLE FOR THE POOR OUTCOME
WHEN THERE IS
A PATIENT DEATH FROM
CONSTIPATION?**

From: McGee, Michael
Sent: Wednesday, June 22, 2016 8:25 AM
Joshua et al.
The capacity to decide who is appropriate
for clozapine or not should be a core
competency for all DSH psychiatrists. If
there are any training issues, then training
should be provided. If there is a need for
feedback, then feedback should be
provided.
I appreciate your question about violence
and clozapine. Many of us, and our patients,
also value the reduction of suffering and
improved functioning that clozapine can
provide. Reduction of violence is not the
only reason to give clozapine. We are also
here to help our patients feelbetter and
function better.
From: Deane, Joshua
Sent: Tuesday, June 21, 2016 4:28 PM
Subject: RE: TRC pre-clozapine
consultation requirement being revisited?

Sure, Dr. Steed, it will be an agenda item for the next Dept. Meeting. I am all for efficiency and cutting through red tape whenever we can, not imposing additional procedure burden on any of our staff. That being said, we also need to be mindful of the fact that yardstick of quality care is not how many of our patients we have managed to put on clozapine. After all, clozapine is no more a panacea than it is a harmless agent.

I don't know whether an increase use of clozapine here in the past 2 years has actually effectuated a tangible reduction of violence in the hospital. (Standards Compliance dept. Should be able to furnish us with some relevant data; and I am going to ask for them just for reference purposes.)

From: Steed, Martin
Sent: Tuesday, June 21, 2016 3:41 PM
Dear Colleagues,
In today's Department of Psychiatry meeting the TRC reported that it was considering reinstating a requirement to obtain a consultation before approving the use of clozapine. This requirement was part

of the reason we only had 30 patients on clozapine 2 years ago whereas
we now have 85. No rationale was given for requiring pre-clozapine consultations other than to presumably control and limit the use of clozapine by DSH-A psychiatrists. I suggest that the
entire Department of Psychiatry be allowed to vote on this matter before our clozapine protocol is changed.
Sincerely,
Staff Psychiatrist
Vice Chief of Staff
Chair: Psychiatry Peer Review and Quality Improvement Committees
From: Cohen, Seth
Sent: Wednesday, June 22, 2016 10:57 AM
This is a meta-analysis and the conclusions should be taken in that light. I do not believe this
can be regarded as a "scholarly challenge" but I appreciate you knowing of this publication.

From: Yee, William
Sent: Wednesday, June 22, 2016 10:55 AM
Efficacy, Acceptability, and Tolerability of Antipsychotics in Treatment-Resistant Schizophrenia:

A Network Meta-analysis
JAMA Psychiatry. 2016;73(3):199-210.
There is definitely a scholarly challenge to
the concept that Clozaril is superior to
other antipsychotics.

From: Cohen, Seth
Sent: Wednesday, June 22, 2016 10:51 AM
I write this somewhat hesitantly as I
understand there are many opinions about
the Clozapine subject and indeed ASH has a
specific, and intense, protocol for dealing
with this special medication. I believe the
most recent data would suggest that
Clozapine has roughly 3% of the
antipsychotic market share in treating
people with schizophrenia. The percentage
of psychiatrists in the US who prescribe
Clozapine (which has been available since
1989) is less than 10%. Certainly there is a
lot of anxiety about prescribing this
somewhat cumbersome agent which
necessitates blood monitoring and a
monitored system which includes the
physician, pharmacy and lab. The data
would suggest that roughly 30% of patients
with schizophrenia indeed have treatment
resistant illness. Clozapine is the only
medication with FDA approved

labeling to treat treatment resistant schizophrenia. The seminal paper (Study 30, published by Kane, Meltzer and Honigfeld in the Archives of General Psychiatry Sept. 1988) clearly notes the efficacy of Clozapine in a truly treatment resistant schizophrenic population. No subsequent study looking at any other antipsychotic (including Olanzapine) in an equally ill treatment resistant group, has ever found an agent with efficacy. Indeed, Clozapine is the "dirtiest drug" known to man. The weight gain and metabolic disturbances are monumental with Clozapine. However, we always weigh risks and benefits. I appreciate the fact that ASH has their Clozapine protocol. I am led to believe that sadly 2 patients at ASH died from Clozapine related GI problems. That cannot be forgotten but should not keep us from using the only FDA approved agent for treatment resistant schizophrenia. I do not know for certain, but well imagine, that ASH has far more than the 90 or so patients on this agent with treatment resistant schizophrenia. In my opinion, certain prescribing practices at ASH are not relective of those in the outside world.

Clozapine can be and is started on treatment resistant patients on an outpatient basis. There is no monitoring of stools, etc. Patients do not routinely die on this agent. I have been prescribing Clozapine dating back to 1986, on a humanitarian protocol basis. I have probably been involved in the care of several hundred patients on Clozapine over the past 30 years. None of my patients died from Clozapine related complications. I have had roughly 5 patients develop agranulocytosis and all of them lived to tell the tale. I had 2 patients develop an ileus with Clozapine, one of whom went for exploratory bowel surgery and similarly lived to tell the tale. I had one patient who developed a pericarditis and survived. I have had at least a dozen patients develop a worsening of their seizure disorders yet this was well managed by the neurologist. Again, this is out of several hundred patients. The benefits of the medication have been relatively monumental, as is routinely described in the literature for decades. The sad reality is that aspirin can lead to bleeding and people have died. That does not mean we should not prescibe aspirin. Anyway, this is a very complex subject but I fear we are making too big of an issue of the whole Clozapine thing and the system may be depriving more of our patients from receiving this special medicine. If there are psychiatrists in our group who are unfamiliar with Clozapine and / or anxious about it, perhaps it would be prudent to think about training all of us so that we do not fear this medicine. I am a newbie here and vow to be a team player so whatever the protocol happens to be, I support it. I do not foresee writing any other such email in the future.

From: Yee, William
Sent: Wednesday, June 22, 2016 12:10 PM
Efficacy, Acceptability, and Tolerability of Antipsychotics in Treatment-Resistant Schizophrenia:
A Network Meta-analysis
JAMA Psychiatry. 2016;73(3):199-210.
We compared the effects of all antipsychotics in patients with treatment-resistant schizophrenia using pairwise meta-analyses and NMA. Olanzapine, clozapine, and risperidone were found to be significantly better than some other antipsychotics in various efficacy outcomes, but the results were not consistent and the

effect sizes were usually small. The most surprising finding was that clozapine was not significantly more efficacious than most other drugs.

Clozapine's superiority was originally demonstrated in a pivotal study5,6 in which it was clearly superior to chlorpromazine in treatment-resistant schizophrenia. Although some subsequent comparisons with FGAs were also statistically significant8,92 and although the superiority to FGAs has been confirmed by meta-analyses,9- 11 the effect size of the original study by Kane et al5,6 (−0.88) has never been replicated. Figure 5 presents the results of all single-comparison clozapine trials5- 8,53,56- 70 and illustrates that, of 21 comparisons, only 2 old studies compared with chlorpromazine,5,6,53 1 study compared with haloperidol,8 and 1 study compared with risperidone56 showed a significant superiority; thus, the failure to find clozapine superior is not an artifact of NMA. The 2 old studies5,6,53 led to a high inconsistency in the NMA, violating a key assumption of the method. We speculate that the inconsistency is in part owing to cohort effects in terms of the periods when these studies were performed because some evidence suggests that the clinical trial quality of psychopharmacologic studies changed significantly after 1990.[89,90] This finding is also evident, among others, by an increasing placebo response[93] and smaller drug-placebo differences.[94,95] Nevertheless, when all trials, irrespective of their publication date, were included, results of the NMA did not substantially differ (eAppendix 6 in the Supplement).

From: Peterson, Richard
Sent: Wednesday, June 22, 2016 11:44 AM
Given that we're an evidence-based group practice, according to a Lancet meta-analysis of 49,000 patients (2013, attached), Clozapine is BY FAR our best agent for therapeutic response in schizophrenia treatment (and violence reduction). If anyone has more credible or specific data, please forward it. As it stands, if we want the best mental health treatment for our severely ill psychotic patients, the data indicates Clozapine is our best option.
From: Peterson, Richard
Sent: Wednesday, June 22, 2016 1:28 PM
Wow, that's helpful, thank you!

From: Yee, William
Sent: Monday, June 27, 2016 9:01 AM
As the individual practitioner I reserve the right to make my decisions based upon my assessment and my clinical experience dating back to 1972.
If the matter is to be determined by a selected knowledgeable committee, then those committee members should be running the Clozaril Clinic and responsible for their decision-making process. Other members of the psychiatric staff should not be responsible for constraints put on them by the committee.

From: Yee, William
Sent: Monday, June 27, 2016 8:57 AM
Efficacy, Acceptability, and Tolerability of Antipsychotics in Treatment-Resistant Schizophrenia:
A Network Meta-analysis
JAMA Psychiatry. 2016;73(3):199-210.
We compared the effects of all antipsychotics in patients with treatment-resistant schizophrenia using pairwise meta-analyses and NMA. Olanzapine, clozapine, and risperidone were found to be significantly better than some other antipsychotics in various efficacy outcomes,

but the results were not consistent and the effect sizes were usually small. The most surprising finding was that clozapine was not significantly more efficacious than most other drugs. Clozapine's superiority was originally demonstrated in a pivotal study5,6 in which it was clearly superior to chlorpromazine in treatment-resistant schizophrenia. Although some subsequent comparisons with FGAs were also statistically significant8,92and although the superiority to FGAs has been confirmed by meta-analyses,9- 11 the effect size of the original study by Kane et al5,6 (−0.88) has never been replicated. Figure 5 presents the results of all single-comparison clozapine trials5- 8,53,56- 70and illustrates that, of 21 comparisons, only 2 old studies compared with chlorpromazine,5,6,53 1 study compared with haloperidol,8 and 1 study compared with risperidone56 showed a significant superiority; thus, the failure to find clozapine superior is not an artifact of NMA. The 2 old studies5,6,53 led to a high inconsistency in the NMA, violating a key assumption of the method. We speculate that the inconsistency is in part owing to cohort effects in terms of the periods when these studies were performed because some evidence suggests that the clinical trial quality of psychopharmacologic studies changed significantly after 1990.89,90 This finding is also evident, among others, by an increasing placebo response93 and smaller drug-placebo differences.94,95 Nevertheless, when all trials, irrespective of their publication date, were included, results of the NMA did not substantially differ (eAppendix 6 in the Supplement).

I will rely on the experts at JAMA to have vetted the article adequately.

I have the patience to wait for future studies to unravel the negative commentary.

I do not believe that this study will be the final study.

I am sure there will be future studies to resolve the disputes.

I will enjoy the outcome, regardless of where it goes.

Will the experts at JAMA be vindicated, or will they be humiliated?

I will not rest my reputation on either side.

I am happy to be a bat on the fence, neither beast nor fowl and without my reputation on the line.

Dr. Yee :)

From: Knapp, Robert
Sent: Monday, June 27, 2016 8:46 AM
Subject: RE: TRC pre-clozapine consultation requirement being revisited?
Coming late to the discussion, but I do want to make the observation that, in the event a patient does not improve in any respect when treated with clozapine, there does not appear to be any good reason to continue it. Let's not continue a treatment if it's not working, just to inflate some numbers.

From: Yee, William
Sent: Monday, June 27, 2016 10:01 AM
We are all credentialled and subject to peer review.
If additional interventions are contemplated and the matter is to be determined by a selected knowledgeable committee, then those committee members should be running the Clozaril Clinic and responsible for their decision-making process.

From: Knapp, Robert
Sent: Monday, June 27, 2016 9:58 AM
I agree, in general. My experience dates back to 1969. However, there are

requirements in law and ethics which limit all of us in our opportunity to practice destructive or "bad" medicine. These limits must be carefully defined and justified, not merely the momentary whim of a "majority."
How to do this? Open to suggestions.

From: Dietch, James
Sent: Wednesday, June 22, 2016 10:19 AM
Surprisingly, Dr. Johnson raises an important issue. Given the complexities of clozapine treatment, it does make sense to utilize an objective rating scale before commiting to such treatment. As many of you are aware, a recent meta-analysis (although met with controversy) challenged the notion that clozapine is the absolute gold standard in psychiatric care. It makes sense for us to objectively rate patients before and after starting clozapine and discontinue treatment if there is no objective benefit. All too often we have seen ineffective treatments continued because we are uncertain what the patient was like before the treatment was started.
If we are to be cutting edge and using clozapine so agressively we should first have in place a mechanism to determine if

the medication has been truly helpful.
Otherwise the risks are not justified.
wE ALSO MAY WANT TO CONSIDER A
CLOZAPINE UNIT. IT WOULD BE MUCH
EASIER TO PLACE A BATHROOM
MONITOR ON ONE UNIT.
I HAVE ALSO BEEN REMINDED
RECENTLY THAT THIS IS A GROUP
PRACTICE.
WHILE THIS IS TRUE, WHO WILL BE
RESPONSIBLE FOR THE POOR OUTCOME
WHEN THERE IS A PATIENT DEATH
FROM CONSTIPATION?

From: Knapp, Robert
Sent: Monday, June 27, 2016 8:56 AM
This is a bigger issue than it may first
appear. Quality of care, appropriate care,
and medically necessary care are not issues
that should be decided by the whim of a
majority vote, but by careful review by a
selected knowledgeable committee with
appropriate training and experience,
and who have the ability to interpret
various contradictory studies, propose and
support justifiable guidelines and
restrictions (if any), and meticulously
document every step of their decision-

making process. Only after deliberation and discussion with the medical staff should a consensus be solicited.

"Pre-Existing text," includes names of symptoms and medical illnesses, medications, people, corporations, law cases, statutes, text of statutes, the titles of articles and books, the content of articles and books cited, FDA Labels and FDA releases and images taken from the internet.

My copyright claim is a claim to the "original text," which is my personal experience as described in the text and my commentary on names of symptoms and medical illnesses, medications, people, corporations, law cases, statutes, text of statutes, the titles of articles and books, the content of articles and books cited, FDA Labels and FDA releases and images taken from the internet.